Essential Oils
For
Hair Growth
Manual

A Step By Step
Guide For
Understanding
Essential Oils

AUTHOR BREANNA RUTTER

TABLE OF CONTENTS

INTRODUCTION TO THE ESSENTIAL OILS FOR HAIR GROWTH MANUAL

"The Essential Oils for Hair Growth Manual is a pocket guide that will provide hair care information and oil recipes that you can formulate in the comforts of your own home to recover from a variety of hair issues! Some of the hair issues that will be discussed in this manual are ways to fix dandruff, thin hair, lice, both forms of alopecia, and so much more! Understanding how long it will take to see desirable results with your hair is dependent upon the natural growth cycle of hair and the severity of your issue as well.

This manual breaks down the hair growth cycle, how much the growth cycle corresponds with your essential oil usage, how to use your recipes, tips on how to distinguish the varying oil qualities, and so much more along the way as you learn how to continue to grow your hair while keeping it in its most healthy state!

When using Essential Oils you are required to be keen to detail to make sure that you are not using essential oils in an inappropriate manner but besides that, treating your hair and scalp is very easy to do. This manual is here to thoroughly educate you about how to use essential oils as well as carrier oils to maintain a healthy scalp and hair.

Please enjoy this informative read, and experiment with a variety of essential oils to achieve your desired results with your hair!"

Sincerely Breanna

1 THE HAIR GROWTH CYCLE

Understanding the life cycle of hair will give you the basic foundation of knowing how long it should take to see results with your hair while using essential oils. Knowing the behavioral characteristics of hair growth will indicate whether or not your hair is responding well to essential oils or if nourishing your hair from the inside is the better option for you (refer to The Dieting For Hair Growth Manual). Understanding how long you should have patience to see desired results with your hair is crucial towards knowing if using essential oils can really make a difference for you!

Hair encounters three stages within its growth/life cycle. Each individual hair growing on your head can be present in different stages of its life cycle and because of that, you lose on average 80 to 100 strands of hair daily. Given that you have on average 100,000 strands of hair on your head, don't be alarmed about shedding because this is a normal process that takes place. Think about it, shed hairs make up way less than 1% of the hair that you have on your scalp right now! Let's discuss the life cycle of hair in further detail.

The Anagen Phase is the 1st phase of the hair life cycle as this is the growing phase because a new hair has begun growing. Since all of your hair is not in the Anagen Phase at once, it will take time before you will notice thickness because other hairs have to enter this phase as well. This phase lasts 2 to 6 years.

The Catagen Phase is the 2nd phase in which your hair is transitioning towards the Telogen phase. The hair is separating from your follicle (see definition guide) and moving upward towards your pore, or the surface of your scalp to fall out as shed hair. This phase lasts 1 to 2 weeks.

The Telogen Phase is the 3rd phase in which the hair is resting because the dermal papilla (see definition guide) separates from the follicle and then moves upward to begin growing a brand new hair. This phase lasts 2 to 4 months.

It is important that you completely understand the growth cycle of hair while using essential oils to yield specific results. The Telogen Phase and the Anagen Phase are the only two phases that allows you to see growth in hair. The time frame between these two phases are 2 months to 6 years. You should not have to wait 6 years to see your hair regrow because remember, all hair is not in the same phase of its life cycle at the same time!

The golden time frame to stick with when trying to obtain results from using essential oils is no longer than 2 to 4 months time to notice desirable changes. You should see changes in as little as 2 months and if you do not see any desirable change, 4 months is the longest time you need to wait to see changes with your hair as a result from using essential oils.

If you have remained consistent in trying a specific oil recommendation (recommendations to be suggested later) and you see no signs of change with your hair within 2 to 4 months, go ahead and try other essential oil recommendations until you find success with achieving hair growth or other desirable changes with your hair!

2 UNDERSTANDING ESSENTIAL OILS

Essential oils are beyond amazing considering the fact that they offer so many healing and therapeutic properties! Essential oils are derived specifically from the peel, flower, bark, and less popularly the seed of any given plant (botanical). Oils derived from the seed of plants are called Carrier Oils and these types of oils will be explained later because their usage is critical towards the delivery of essential oils!

Essential oils are extracted from plants through a process called distillation (refer to the definition guide). These oils are volatile (evaporates easily) and without proper storage, sunlight and exposure to air will oxidize causing it to reduce in its potency.

These oils carry their scent which makes them perfect for aromatherapy. Different essential oils can improve your mood by eliminating depression or anxiety, can induce sleepiness for those who struggle with insomnia and even improves alertness as well.

Essential oils are able to penetrate deeply into your body improving your skin and hair and are widely used for treating a variety of hair issues! These oils stimulate your sebaceous gland (refer to the definition guide) which is great for your hair. Depending on what kind of hair issues you face, certain oils will diminish dandruff, stimulate scalp blood flow, create shinier hair, soothe eczema or psoriasis, unclog your pores, soften hair, and stimulate your hair follicles for growth and strength which is desired by many!

Additionally, essential oils can pose a risk to those who are pregnant, suffering from high blood pressure or epilepsy. Please consult with your doctor before using essential oils!

3 UNDERSTANDING CARRIER OILS

Carrier oils are derived from the seeds of plants since seeds contain the large percentage of fats. Carrier oils yield more yield more oil from the plant than the yield of essential oils and that is why carrier oils (oils like almond, olive, coconut etc.) are able to be sold in larger containers and quantities while essential oils are sold in smaller containers and in lower quantities. Also, omega fats are predominately found in the seeds or nuts of plants (and also in fish) such as Omega 3,6 and 9. Omega 9 benefits your health but Omega 3 and Omega 6 are the only omega fats that can interfere with the production of DHT (Dihydrotestosterone) which causes hair loss. So if you are suffering from hair loss or thinning, increase your intake of Omega 3 and 6 fats! Let's discuss in further detail how carrier oils are extracted and their differences in quality.

Carrier oils "carry" essential oils and other nutrients to your body whether you use them topically or ingest them orally. Some individuals like to ingest a low dosage of essential oils with distilled water to benefit the body but to contribute specifically to the growth and health of your hair, essential oils should be applied to the surface of the skin!

Carrier oils can be cold pressed or expeller pressed and unrefined or refined.

Cold pressed oils are pressurized and heated with temperatures below 120-150° to help extract the oil while also retaining all of its nutritional value.

Expeller pressed oils are pressurized and heated to temperatures over 150° to extract the oil and this causes the oil to lose some nutritional value.

Unrefined oils are no longer treated passed being pressed and this can result in either a cold pressed unrefined oil or an expeller pressed unrefined oil.

Refined oils have been bleached and/or deodorized to eliminate color and/or fragrance. This results in either cold pressed refined oils or expeller pressed refined oils. From the most nutritional oil quality to least goes as listed;

Cold Pressed Unrefined Oil
Expeller Pressed Unrefined Oil
Cold Pressed Refined Oil
Expeller Pressed Unrefined Oil

Cold Pressed Unrefined Oils are the best carrier oils to use topically (and in conjunction with essential oils) for your hair and scalp because this quality of oil provides the highest potency of nutritional value that an oil can possess. Some individuals do not like the naturally occurring fragrance of the oil in this quality, so a refined version instead is better for some, even if it contains a lower nutritional value.

Virgin Oil and Extra Virgin Oil are terms usually describe whether or not an oil is cold pressed or expeller pressed and least commonly, referenced to whether or not your oil of choice is blended with other oils or if it is 100% a specific oil of choice. Virgin Oils are expeller pressed or can contain a blend of oils and Extra Virgin Oils are cold pressed or contain 100% of a specific oil. Many debate about whether or not these terms are a play on words because they aren't consistently labeled accordingly. The best way to determine the equality of your carrier oil is to read the ingredients list and description of the product. The highest quality of oil should be 100% (your carrier oil of choice) Cold Pressed and Unrefined!

4 OILS FOR HAIR GROWTH

When choosing essential oils and carrier oils for hair growth, you have to look for two unique qualities these oils possess such as the ability to increase blood flow and stimulate the dermal papilla (refer to the definition guide).

ESSENTIAL OILS FOR HAIR GROWTH
Rosemary, Cedarwood, Thyme, Peppermint, Spearmint, Lavender and Mustard Essential Oil

CARRIER OILS FOR HAIR GROWTH
Olive, Vitamin E, Emu and Carrot Oil

OIL RECIPES FOR HAIR GROWTH

(Recipes are created based on how well the scents complement one another)

Rosemary Oil Blend

3 drops of Rosemary Essential Oil
1 drop of Cedarwood Essential Oil
1 drop of Thyme Essential Oil
1 ounce (2 tbsp.) of Olive Oil

Peppermint Oil Blend

3 drops of Peppermint Essential Oil
3 drops of Spearmint Essential Oil
1 ounce (2 tbsp.) of Vitamin E Oil

5 OILS FOR AREATA & TRACTION ALOPECIA

When choosing essential oils and carrier oils to treat areata alopecia and traction alopecia, you have to look for unique qualities these oils possess such as the ability to increase blood flow, stimulate the dermal papilla (refer to the definition guide) and is high in Omega 3 and Omega 6 fats.

ESSENTIAL OILS FOR
AREATA AND TRACTION ALOPECIA
Saw Palmetto, Stinging Nettle, Burdock Root, Peppermint and Cypress Essential Oil

CARRIER OILS FOR
AREATA AND TRACTION ALOPECIA
Safflower and Castor Oil

OIL RECIPE FOR
AREATA & TRACTION ALOPECIA

(Recipes are created based on how well the scents complement one another)

Saw Palmetto Oil Blend

3 drops of Saw Palmetto Essential Oil
2 drops of Stinging Nettle Essential Oil
1 drop of Burdock Root
1 ounce (2 tbsp.) of Safflower Oil

6 OILS TO THICKEN HAIR

When choosing essential oils and carrier oils to thicken thin hair, look for unique qualities these oils possess such as the ability to retain or add protein to thicken hair that is fine no matter if your hair is thick or thin. Refer to the definition guide to understand the differences between these types of hair!

ESSENTIAL OILS FOR THICKENING HAIR
Lavender and Ylang Ylang Essential Oil

CARRIER OILS FOR THICKENING HAIR
Castor, Coconut, Jamaican Black Castor and Grass Fed Oil

OIL RECIPES TO THICKEN HAIR

(Recipes are created based on how well the scents complement one another)

Lavender Oil Blend

6 drops of Lavender Essential Oil
1 tbsp. of Castor Oil
1 tbsp. of Coconut Oil

Ylang Ylang Oil Blend

6 drops of Ylang Ylang Essential Oil
1 ounce (2 tbsp.) of Grass Fed Butter

(Jamaican Black Castor Oil can be used alone!)

7 OILS FOR STRONGER HAIR

When choosing essential oils and carrier oils to make weak hair stronger, you have to look for unique qualities these oils possess such as the ability to retain or add protein similar to the oils for thickening hair. Additionally, your oils need to have the ability to strengthen hair by increasing its elasticity. The more flexible your hair, the stronger it becomes!

ESSENTIAL OILS FOR STRONGER HAIR
Bay and Ylang Ylang Essential Oil

CARRIER OILS FOR STRONGER HAIR
Argan, Sesame, Coconut, Castor and Avocado Oil

OIL RECIPES FOR STRONGER HAIR

(Recipes are created based on how well the scents complement one another)

Bay Oil Blend

6 drops of Bay Essential Oil
1 tbsp. of Argan Oil
1 tbsp. of Avocado Oil

Ylang Ylang Oil Blend

6 drops of Ylang Ylang Essential Oil
1 tbsp. of Sesame Oil
1 tbsp. of Coconut Oil

8 OILS FOR DANDRUFF CONTROL

Many essential oils by default, stimulate your sebaceous glands (refer to definition guide) which increase your sebum production while offering anti-septic qualities. There are a special set of essential oils and carrier oils that are superior in its effects to do both of these things simultaneously which makes them an excellent natural remedy for curing dandruff and even dry scalp! Regulating your sebum production is the first step towards ridding dandruff!

ESSENTIAL OILS FOR DANDRUFF
Tea Tree, Lemon, Clary Sage, Myrrh and Lavender
Essential Oil

CARRIER OILS FOR DANDRUFF
Grapeseed, Jojoba Oil and Almond Oil

OIL RECIPES FOR DANDRUFF CONTROL

Tea Tree Oil Blend

4 drops of Tea Tree Essential Oil
2 drops of Lemon Essential Oil
1 ounce (2 tbsp.) of Grapeseed Oil

Clary Sage Oil Blend

4 drops Clary Sage Essential Oil
2 drops Myrrh Essential Oil
1 ounce (2 tbsp.) of Jojoba Oil

9 OILS FOR ITCHY SCALP

When choosing essential oils and carrier oils to cater to an itchy scalp, you have to look for unique qualities these oils possess such as the ability to soothe and tighten your scalp pores to prevent irritation. Using oils that mimic your natural sebum secretion (like jojoba oil) is the best when keeping your scalp moisturized!

ESSENTIAL OILS FOR ITCHY SCALP
Rose, Myrrh, Lemon, Lavender, and Tea Tree Essential Oil

CARRIER OILS FOR ITCHY SCALP
Jojoba and Grapeseed Oil

OIL RECIPES FOR ITCHY SCALP

Rose Oil Blend

3 drops of Rose Essential Oil
2 drops of Myrrh Essential Oil
1 drop of Lemon Essential Oil
1 ounce (2 tbsp.) of Jojoba Oil

Lavender Oil Blend

3 drops of Lavender Essential Oil
3 drops of Tea Tree Essential Oil
1 ounce (2 tbsp.) of Grapeseed Oil

10 OILS FOR INFLAMMATION

When choosing essential oils and carrier oils to calm an inflamed scalp, some of the essential oils will be similar to treating an itchy scalp because you will need something that soothes your irritated skin. Carrier oils high in omega fats are important for protecting your hair and also nourishing for your skin with vital fats that will also lock in moisture. The suggested recipes are perfect for those who suffer from scalp conditions like eczema and psoriasis for example.

ESSENTIAL OILS FOR INFLAMMATION
Chamomile, Sandalwood, Eucalyptus, Tea Tree, Clary Sage, Bergamot, Patchouli, Helichrysum, Burdock and Neroli Essential Oil

CARRIER OILS FOR INFLAMMATION
Olive, Apricot, Marula, Avocado, Jojoba, Tamanu and Castor Oil

---

OIL RECIPES FOR INFLAMMATION

Chamomile Oil Blend

5 drops of Chamomile Essential Oil
1 tbsp. of Olive Oil
1 tbsp. of Apricot Oil

Sandalwood Oil Blend

3 drops of Sandalwood Essential Oil
2 drops of Eucalyptus Essential Oil
1 ounce (2 tbsp.) of Marula Oil

---

11 OILS FOR LICE TREATMENT

Lice are horrible parasites and a pain to get rid of but with a potent concoction of essential oils and carrier oils, those bugs don't stand a chance! Lice hate citrus oils (since they are high in acidity) and also heavier oils make it harder for them to live comfortable on your scalp. After applying your oil recipe, leave it on the scalp and cover it overnight with a plastic shower cap. In the morning, comb through your hair with a fine tooth comb and follow up with a shampoo wash. This may take a couple of treatments to become a 100% lice free!

ESSENTIAL OILS FOR LICE TREATMENT
Lemon, Lemon Grass Oil, Roman Chamomile, German Chamomile and Geranium Essential Oil

CARRIER OILS FOR LICE TREATMENT
Olive and Sesame Oil

OIL RECIPES FOR LICE TREATMENT

Lemon Oil Blend
3 drops of Lemon Essential Oil
2 drops of Lemongrass Essential Oil
1 drop of Roman Chamomile
1 ounce (2 tbsp.) Sesame Oil

German Chamomile Oil Blend
4 drops of German Chamomile Essential Oil
2 drops of Geranium Essential Oil
1 ounce (2 tbsp.) of Olive Oil

AFTERWORDS

"This manual of course was made in mind for those who desire to know how to use essential oils for the benefit of healthy hair and/or a healthy scalp. As you may have read throughout these chapters, this manual is condensed with priceless information for helping you successfully recover from a lot of unfortunate situations with your hair. You may have chosen to read this guide because you support my work, you were looking for information on using Essential Oils, or you were looking for this information to help a loved one.

Personally, I have never used essential oils for the purpose of benefiting my hair and scalp but I have used hair care products before in the past that contained small traces of essential oils. I do not believe that those small amount of essential oils lead to the health of my hair because the health of my hair has been consistently maintained by keeping my scalp and hair cleansed and most importantly, sealing moisture into my hair with an oil sealant of choice. Using essential oils for hair care is a staple for many DIY (do it yourself) individuals who want to control every aspect of their hair care products, at least to the degree of restoring the health of their hair or scalp.

I hope that you thoroughly enjoyed this read, it was a pleasure of mine to write this for your knowledge and enjoyment." Sincerely, Breanna

ADDITIONAL RESOURCES

The Official Website: www.Howtoblackhair.com

The Online Store: www.HowtoblackhairStore.com

Free Subscription Email: http://eepurl.com/FZs5b

For Additional Hair Questions

YourHairQuestions@Gmail.com

Black Hair Styling Tutorials

BlackWomenHair YouTube Channel

www.Youtube.com/BlackWomenHair

HowToBlackHair YouTube Channel

www.Youtube.com/HowToBlackHair

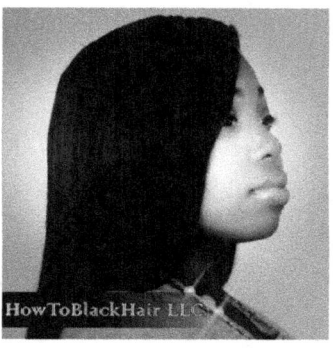

The Natural Hair Bible

The 10 Commandments of Black Hair Care

www.HowToBlackHair.com

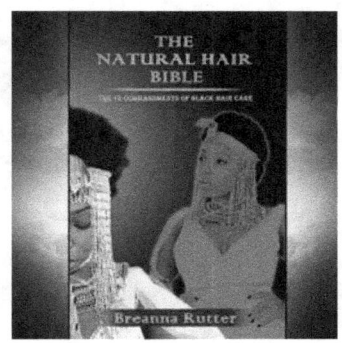

The Relaxed Hair Bible

The 10 Commandments of Long Healthy Relaxed Hair

www.HowToBlackHair.com

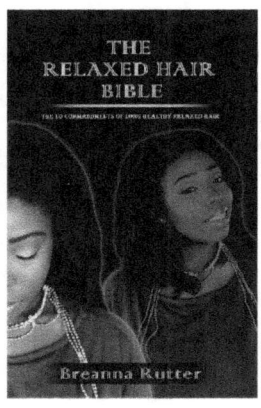

Black Hair Styling DVDs (Over 20+ Hairstyles)

www.HowToBlackHair.com

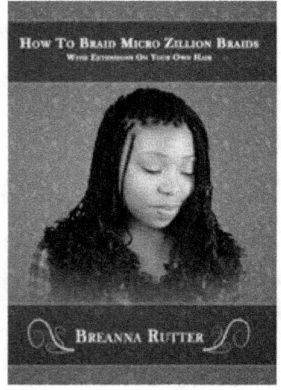 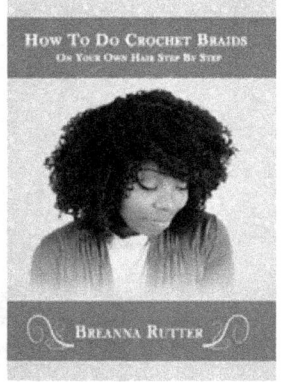

DEFINITION GUIDE

Antiseptic: *a substance that can revert the growth of a disease causing organism*

Areata Alopecia: *random hair loss triggered by your immune system*

Aromatherapy: *using fragrant plant extracts to cause mental or physical improvements*

Botanical: *obtaining substance from plants to be used as an ingredient in other products*

Dermal Papilla: *a raised dermis located underneath the root of your follicle that houses the blood supply*

DHT(Dihydrotestosterone): *an enzyme that develops with the conversion of testosterone and Type II 5-alpha reductase, which is located in the oil gland of your hair follicle*

Distillation: *extracting the essential of a plant through the action of heating a cooling the liquid substance*

Elasticity: *the stretching ability of your hair*

Fine Hair: *your individual strands of hair are closer in size (circumference) to string instead of thread*

Hair Follicles: *an individual strand of hair*

Oxidize: *a substance that evaporates by becoming chemically bound to oxygen*

Sebaceous Gland: *a small gland underneath your skin that secretes an oil called sebum to lubricate and protect your hair and scalp*

Sebum: *the oil that secretes from your sebaceous gland*

Thick Hair: *your ponytail width, with all of your hair gathered, is the width of a quarter or larger*

Thin Hair: *your ponytail width, with all of your hair gathered, is the width of a nickel or smaller*

Traction Alopecia: *gradual hair loss usually caused by a pulling force on your hair from hair styling*

Volatile: *a substance evaporates with ease even while at a normal room temperate*

INDEX

HOW TO BLACK HAIR LLC.
WRITTEN BY BREANNA RUTTER
BOOK DESIGNED BY BREANNA RUTTER
COVER DESIGNED BY JARED RUTTER
ALL RIGHTS RESERVED.
VISIT WWW.HOWTOBLACKHAIR.COM

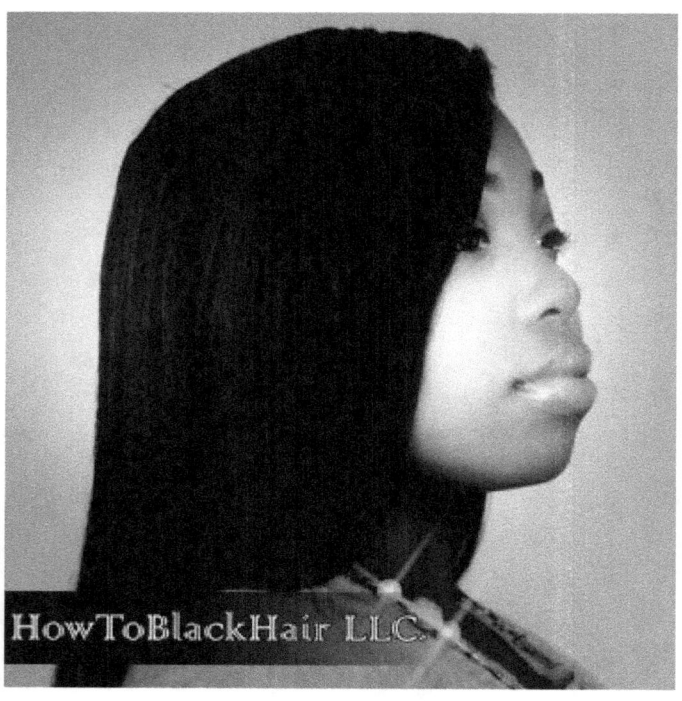

www.ingramcontent.com/pod-product-compliance
Lightning Source LLC
Chambersburg PA
CBHW070254290526
45789CB00004B/1844